For Kelly...
Who shows her support
for me in a thousand ways

Weighing In
On the big problem

*Seven Pillars of information and encouragement you
need to lose weight and keep it off!*

By Mark Gerard

Table of contents

Introduction

Chapter one
My personal battle

Are you healthy enough to lose weight?

Determination, Keep a sense of humor

Chapter two
Fat, Calories, Protein, Carbs & Fiber

Chapter three
Taking a free day

Accountability and honesty

Things that help

Chapter four
The spice of life

Chapter five
The Weigh In program

Questions and answers

Vocabulary and Definitions

Suggested Menus

Final thoughts

Bibliography

About the author

*Introduction

Since you are reading this book, there is no doubt that you want to lose weight. You have probably tried many fad diets and even gimmicks, but here you are; maybe even a bit frustrated. Maybe this is your "last effort". So, first things first: let me be clear, that this book "**Weighing In** on the big problem" is not a diet plan. It is not a sales pitch to get you to buy a lot of products and it is not a gimmick.

Weighing In is a safe, carefully thought out life style change. It is a deliberate decision to make changes that will help you lose weight and improve your health in the process. The goal is to show you how and where you can make these changes, to help you reach your personal goal in weight loss and, as a bonus, to be healthier and happier than before you started.

CHAPTER ONE

*My personal battle

I remember several times over the past few years looking at and reading materials on diets and weight loss, even exercise for that matter, and the person who spoke or wrote looked to be about 21 years old and probably never had more than five pounds to lose. In the back of my mind I was thinking "you know, I looked that good when I was in my twenties too." But I'm not 21 years old anymore, yet I find myself wanting to look and feel good again. More important than that, I want to be healthy!

The simple truth is that about six months before I really found the determination and the encouragement to lose weight **I was around a hundred pounds overweight**. I found a "weigh-in" chart I made, and my weight was 287 pounds (130 kilos).

Somehow, even with the information that I was more than a hundred pounds overweight, it took me another six months to say to myself "enough is enough".

Now, I have made New Year's resolutions before, and broken them. I said it was time to trim down, and then didn't. I began exercise programs that yielded some fruit, but didn't last more than five or six weeks at best. And yes, I tried the fads, celebrity diets, and I even tried "a cleanse".

My personal battle with weight took me through a symphony of emotions, struggles and self-defeating attitudes. It was a rollercoaster of poor choices, discouraging moments, and too much work with too little rest.

The good news is this: I took off the weight and I have kept it off. And you can too! What's more interesting is that I didn't take any "weight-loss" pills, I didn't drink any shakes, and I didn't join any programs. No crazy gym workouts, no food sent to my home. Just doing what I have come to call my "**Weigh In**" program.

Are you healthy enough to lose weight?

I laughed the first time I saw a commercial for one of those erectile dysfunction drugs... it said, something like this:"check with your physician to be sure you're healthy enough to have sex"; yeah, right. As if the answer would change the decision.

So, it seems strange to say that you should speak with your family doctor to be sure you're healthy enough to lose weight! **Do it anyway.** *Let your doctor know that you want to do light exercise and eat better, with the goal of losing weight and living healthier. At the very least, you will really make his day.*

Determination

I have found that there is no stopping a determined person. Years ago I took a "language aptitude" test which indicated that I was not likely to ever learn a foreign language. What the test could not measure was my determination. Today I speak four languages and I'm helping my wife learn her fifth language, which is her way of spurring me on.

Your determination to lose weight and live healthy is vital. No one else can "want it for you" or "do it for you".... You must want it for yourself! It helps to have a "never give up" attitude, and in this case, it makes a huge difference.

Make no mistake about it, if you are not determined, you will not lose weight regardless of the plan you follow. The **Weigh In** *program is more of a life style change; you won't be hungry following it, but you will have to be determined to stay away from certain foods... that is if you can refer to highly processed "fake food" as food.*

*Keep a sense of humor

+Laughter – like medicine. "A merry heart does good like medicine." Proverbs 17:22. It is possible, with weight loss, like most things in life, to take yourself too seriously. To be determined is one thing, but learn to laugh. Learn the art of being happy. Personally, I laugh at myself all the time.

Health Guidance.org points out what God's Word told us thousands of years ago, that laughter is like medicine. You see, laughter releases endorphins that cause you to feel better and even help against depression.

You need to understand something: emotions play a role in weight loss! Negative emotions can have adverse effects on your health as well as your weight. Positive emotions, like a sense of humor and laughter, can have a good effect. Why not take advantage of every tool in the weight loss toolbox? Laugh!

CHAPTER TWO

*The role of Fat, Calories, Protein, Carbohydrates and Fiber

Let's consider the fat in our diet

Over the years we have all heard a lot about eating low-fat, fat-free, low cholesterol and reducing calories, so much so that I personally felt that I'd go crazy if I heard another study about how something natural (like eggs) was causing problems today, but our parents and grandparents never had a problem with it.

There are, however a few basics that are important, and they can help you have success. First, remember that **there are good fats and bad fats**. Natural fats found in real food are not the enemy. For example: the fat found in avocados is not only natural, but extremely good for you. You never want to eliminate these good fats. If you are only cutting fats in general, you could be permitting bad fats while eliminating good ones. However, the fats found in what I call "fake food" or processed foods are to be strictly limited or eliminated from your daily diet. If you have to open a package or a can, you can be sure you're consuming a lot of things you don't need, fat among them. These "fake foods" are not only loaded with fat,

Cut out the man-made packaged fats and keep the natural, good fats found in real foods.

but can also contain enormous amounts of salt and sugar, not to mention preservatives and additives you would never add to your foods while cooking at home. The same is true with packaged products labeled as "low-fat" or "fat-free"; they are not healthy for you in any way, and are usually loaded with modified wheat flour, sugar and other ingredients that hinder weight less efforts. If you are only **obsessed with dietary fat**, then you are overlooking other extremely important factors. Cut out the man-made packaged fats and keep the natural, good fats found in real foods.

NOT ALL CALORIES AFFECT
US THE SAME WAY!

Take a closer look at calories

I want to talk about **calories** *for a moment. Many people have been taught that all you have to do is count calories and you will lose weight. I am sure, however, that it has not escaped you that some people count their calories and lose a lot, while others lose little or nothing at all. Do you want to know why? It's simple: not all calories affect us the same. Let me give you an example: one slice of white bread has 76 calories. One scrambled egg with milk has 101 calories.* **So, if all you looked at was the calorie count***, you might believe the white bread (or toast) might be a better choice. The thing is, the bread has a Glycemic Index, which we'll look at shortly, that is off the charts; it's loaded with carbohydrates, and is made from modified and processed wheat, all of which affect our bodies negatively; so if you ate the bread (or toast) you would have consumed fewer calories, but it would not be the best choice in so many other ways. Let me say again that not all calories affect us the same. Let's look at the calories, for instance, from a bagel vs. the calories from a steak. A plain 3 ½ inch bagel has about 195 calories . Six ounces of beef would have about 500 calories. The bagel however will have a negative effect on blood sugar levels, whereas the beef will not.*

Do not worry about calories, as we will take them into account for you, but this program looks at them in a completely different light.

Protein must be considered as well

Consider **protein** *a moment. The body needs proteins for just about everything that goes on; building muscle, skin, hair, organs, not to mention that our immune system needs antibodies which are made by proteins. Our hormones as well as metabolism, need proteins: those amino acids or smaller molecules that make up proteins.*

We usually think of meat when protein is mentioned. However, protein can be found in both plant and animal food sources.

Carbohydrates

We must examine **carbohydrates***. First of all you need to know that there are two types of Carbohydrates or carbs: simple carbs and complex carbs. Think about sugars and starches, because these are the most common and most readily available carbs. The sugars will represent our simple carbs, which are absorbed into the blood stream very quickly. Starches, grains and vegetables will represent our complex carbs, which are broken down much slower and therefore do not affect blood sugar levels the same. Another way you can divide carbs into two categories is: healthy and unhealthy. The healthy carbs would be derived from non- processed foods, like fruit, vegetables and beans, while the unhealthy carbs would come from processed, refined and packaged foods containing white flour and sugar.*

The highly processed, refined and packaged foods, where we find most of the unhealthy carbohydrates, are a chief contributor to diabetes and heart disease not to mention obesity.

Remember that I said "not all calories affect us the same"? Well, calories from unhealthy carbohydrates are a good example, like candy bars and other types of processed snacks; and they generally consist of sugar of one type or another.

The Glycemic Index

You may not have heard much about **the Glycemic Index (GI)** *so let me give you a condensed lesson. I've placed this information under the carbohydrate section because the G I is in fact a numerical index that ranks carbs based on their conversion to glucose (simple sugar) in the human body. Perhaps what is most important about the GI is that your body does its best* work *when the blood sugar is kept somewhat constant; levels that are either too low or too high cause problems that can be avoided. So understanding this Index can be helpful.*

The Glycemic Index helps you evaluate what is a complex carb vs what might be a simple carb. And as I mentioned before, complex carbs move into the blood stream slower, while simple carbs go quickly.

Not all experts are agreed as to the value and accuracy of the GI, and while some good studies have been done, there is a lot of work ahead before we understand everything we need to know to really take advantage of the Glycemic Index.

Take a good look at Fiber

Consider **fiber**. This little guy is interesting, because fiber is a type of carbohydrate, but one that the body cannot digest. So it passes through the body undigested and helps to regulate such things as blood sugar levels as well as keeping hunger at distance.

Fiber is only found in our food supply from the earth, or plants. There are two types of fiber: insoluble and soluble. Both are needed for healthy living. Like water, most people do not get enough fiber in their diet either. So, the more you understand about nutrition, and in this case, fiber, the easier you will find it to stay with the **Weigh In** program and reach your goal.

*Your success: the frustration of family and friends

+Not everyone wants to know. The fact is, this drives our friends and family crazy. Be careful that your success with weight loss doesn't drive everyone away.

Like our faith, weight loss is best not shoved into the faces of others. Listen to me, our friends and family have eyes; they can see. They might even comment or ask a question, and when they do it is okay to answer or respond, short and sweet, and then drop the subject. We often spend time visiting while we eat; which is not a good time to talk about losing weight.

+No one wants to hear about it 24/7. It is easy to "overload" the ones around us with what we're doing, but no one *wants to hear about it all the time, in fact, take my word for it, they may not want to hear about it at all!*

When those who really do want to talk to you about your success with weight loss come asking, take the time away from the crowd and give them the same resources, information and encouragement that helped you, but don't do it over a meal, make it an appointment for coffee.

CHAPTER THREE

Taking a "free day"

A hard truth that I've learned along the way is that it is not a good idea to follow a healthy plan for exercise and eating and then take the weekend off. You know what I mean by taking a day or the weekend off, right? I'm talking about having a "buffet mentality". That is eating what you want, how you want it. Don't worry about exercise today, because you will be back with the "program" on Monday.

**This is the hard place where many people just give up...
But I suspect that since you're reading this book, you want a change.**

Here is the problem with such a plan, and while I'm sharing this with you, know that I have literally lived this. I can best explain the problem with the well-known cruise ship passenger weight gain. The average passenger on a cruise ship gains seven to ten pounds during a week-long cruise! Ouch, ten pounds in just a week!

Now think about how long it takes you to lose just 2 pounds. If you successfully lose 2 pounds a week, such weight gain would **set you back 5 weeks**, not to mention the discouragement you will feel.

This is the hard place where many people just give up. Then they begin to think, and later to say, "Oh, it's my metabolism", "I'm big boned" or "It's genetic".

You have probably been there. Maybe you're there now. But I suspect that since you're reading this book, **you want a change.**

My wife calls it "sabotage". You know, something done that will cause failure. That is what taking a weekend off or even an entire day off can do to you. You need to think about it in smaller terms. Instead of allowing yourself to indulge in the same habits that caused you to gain weight, allow yourself some of whatever it is that temps you; say, your favorite pie or cheesecake. (Sorry, I'm not trying to make you hungry) ☺ Now, cut the portion in half, set it away from you, and enjoy a little bit of a treat. **Right now you can't do that**, but later, if you're careful, you can from time to time. One of the weight loss commercials said, "We're not gonna give up what we love". This "slogan" will not help you. There are a lot of processed carbohydrates that we should give up, or at least learn to avoid most of the time, if not all the time.

You're dedicated efforts to get your body into a fat burning mode do not need to be "turned off" every weekend

My weight gain happened gradually over twenty years. To stay focused and committed to reaching my goal for just one year, after twenty years of neglect was a small sacrifice compared to the life-long benefits. You may not need to lose 100 pounds, but whether you want to lose 30 pounds or 50 pounds, you will have greater success if you avoid the free days; but be warned, neither **Weigh In** nor any other program will help you if you want a free day every time you turn around.

What's more, you'll regret the moments of weakness, and the after affects last longer than the momentary, false pleasures. You're dedicated efforts to get your body into a fat burning mode do not need to be "turned off" every weekend.

*Accountability and honesty

No one wants to talk about being overweight, or about obesity. The thing is, we don't even want to talk about it with ourselves. Listen to me: that will not work. In order to make a change in your life that has the end result of weight loss and healthier living, you need to start by being honest with yourself. It was nice to think that the absence of visible medical problems or undiagnosed medical conditions meant that I was in good health. That just is not the truth.

*My story is one of silence and denial. Inside I was wondering how a kid could go from setting the quarter mile record in high school to being overweight? How did an Air Force vet that used to run six miles several times a week get to be fat? In case you haven't noticed, I didn't use the word "obese" when speaking about weight, that is, **until I got honest with myself!** You see…*

The absence of visible medical problems or undiagnosed medical conditions does not constitute good health!

Things that help!

Now there are things that I did that truly helped me a great deal. The lack of these made a difference in my past failures, and the inclusion of these things helped me experience success as I learned to take advantage of them. They will help you too.

+Admitting I had a problem. In particular I needed to admit that I was a **carbohydrate addict**. *It is believed that about 75% of overweight people and many normal weight people are carbohydrate addicts. This is not an imagined or made up addiction. Dr. Oz and many other authorities have addressed this problem. This addiction often triggers* **hypoglycemia**, *which has symptoms of shakiness, sweating, irritability intense cravings etc… Carbohydrate addicts tend to know that something is different with the way their bodies respond to snacks, starches, desserts and junk food. The consumption of refined carbohydrates can and often does lead to serious health problems including obesity and type two diabetes which can affect both your quality of life as well as your length of life. It is sad how the sale and consumption of flour and sugar have* become so acceptable in western society. Even the USDA recommends that more than half our diet should consist of carbohydrates. Never mind that there are doctors who believe that carbohydrate addiction rivals that of cocaine, only worse, because it messes with your metabolism as well as your neurological system. You must deal with this addiction so that you can have success in this area.

You need to confront your carbohydrate addiction in order to start on the road

to weight loss and a life change

+ *A food journal or log helped me. Personally I resisted keeping a journal / log because I wanted to cheat a little. Naturally, that's what gets us all into trouble. It was the combination of my desire to cheat a little and my forgetfulness that set me up for failure. Keeping an honest log of everything that goes into your mouth will help you not sabotage your own goals and hard work. In the back of the book I've included the logs I used. You don't need to buy anything, or even print these logs. You may prefer to keep your log on your phone, kindle or tablet. There are some great apps available these days. Also, keep a file of your logs, I'd say a month's worth anyway. This is important so that you can review what you've done right or where you need to do better. One last thing, if you have special circumstances, a special event, dinner at a friend's home or a long drive, note that in the margin of your log sheet, it can help you as well because such changes and meals that are out of your control do affect your progress.*

+*The scale helped me. My wife and my mother taught me this. The scale isn't something to be afraid of, but rather it is your faithful, truthful friend.*

*A good weight scale to monitor your steps and successes is absolutely essential. While you don't need to invest a great deal of money to use the **"Weigh in"** program that helped me lose 100 lbs., buying a good scale is one of the best weight loss investments you can make for your own health and that of your family.*

Now, don't go to the store and buy the cheapest one available. Look for a scale in between the cheapest and the costliest, and you'll do alright. I'm deliberately not mentioning a brand name or pushing a certain company. My goal is not to push you to buy other products. (I feel the same way about recommending supplements and other items). Use it! Weigh in, and log it; and try and weigh in more or less the same time every day. In the morning after you have gone to the bathroom might be the easiest.

+My clothes helped me. Our appearance and the way our clothes fit and feel are a good indicator of our weight and/or change in weight.

I was really looking forward to buying some nice, new clothes, but I was disgusted with myself when the first 20 pounds I lost only resulted in me properly fitting into the clothes I was already wearing. Your spouse and friends might not tell you the hard truth, but your clothes will.

+The mirror helped me. Clearly the mirror can be painfully honest. That's not a bad thing, because each week you will be able to notice a difference. Like the scale, don't avoid using the full length mirror. "Mirror, mirror on the wall…"

CHAPTER FOUR

*The Spice of life

Spices are such a blessing in this world. They add so much to the flavor of our food, but did you know that spices do so much more? Antioxidant power is chief among the health benefits. Antioxidants are nutrients and enzymes that help prevent the occurrence of chronic diseases like heart disease and cancer, just to name a couple. Antioxidants can offer protection against illnesses like stroke, arthritis and other diseases.

Spices also offer benefits toward weight loss, among other things, **boosting metabolism**. We want to boost our metabolism! And we know that spices have anti-inflammatory properties that are really beneficial in so many ways like calming or even eliminating arthritis.

The topic of spices could have its own book, so space will not allow me to do more than touch on the subject. Let me mention just a few: Cinnamon; Garlic; Paprika; Oregano; Chili peppers; Parsley; Thyme; Rosemary, Ginger; Anise; Basil; Cayenne; Celery seed; Cilantro; Mustard; Onion; Sage; Jalapeños; Turmeric; and don't forget Salt and Pepper. These spices should be included in your food. You can put them in either your coffee or tea or your food in general. Some spices are also used as topical creams. Let us use every tool available in the weight loss tool box.

*What about supplements or vitamins?

When you begin to burn the fat reserves and start losing weight, it will be like your car using a low grade fuel source: which is just what fat is. Sometimes you put an additive into the fuel tank to *help your car use that low grade fuel. Well, our bodies can use supplements while we're burning off all those fat reserves.*

Your body's functions: appetite, hunger, metabolic rate, metabolism of fats and sugars, and calorie-burning, work more efficiently when it has the ideal consumption of vitamins and minerals.

*I believe that the healthiest way for you to consume vitamins and minerals is through the consumption of the real foods you eat. However, when a person is over-weight, the body is not functioning correctly. This metabolic imbalance needs to be corrected and supplements can assist you in this process. Flax seed, for example, is excellent for our heart health. It contains both omega 3 and omega 6, as well as omega 9. There is a study by Weston Price that found that vitamin A is essential for our bodies to be able to make use of all other vitamins and minerals in our system. You do want / need to get enough fiber in your diet, and there are several rich in fiber foods you should consider, and psyllium husks are helpful if you need additional fiber in your diet. The large family of B vitamins is extremely important in many ways, but perhaps the most important for you right now is the fact that **this family of vitamins helps us with metabolism**. If you are not eating enough foods rich in vitamin B, you should consider this supplement as well. Additionally, because vitamin B is a water-soluble vitamin, which means that it is not stored in the body but needs a daily supply, this needs your attention.*

Your first goal should be to try and get the vitamins and minerals that you need through the real foods you consume. If you need to buy vitamins and mineral supplements, be sure to purchase good quality products.

CHAPTER FIVE

The "Weigh In" Program

*Now, let me share with you about how the "**Weigh In**" program works. As I do this, you will be able to see how it grew from a simple diet into a lifestyle change for me.*

In principle, our bodies use the food we eat to produce the energy we need. When we eat, if the "fuel" we put in is not used, it is then stored, usually as fat. Everyone knows that sugar, for example, gives you an instant burst of energy; as do many similar carbohydrates. Your metabolism is burning the carbs you're consuming, and then storing what is not needed at that moment.

But what happens if you force your body to burn fat reserves instead of the "instant energy" found in processed carbohydrates? Well, simply put, you lose weight. Is that possible? Absolutely.

*The **Weigh In** program is designed to help your body change from living from carb to carb while burning carbs from frequent consumption, to using and burning fat reserves which leads to weight loss.*

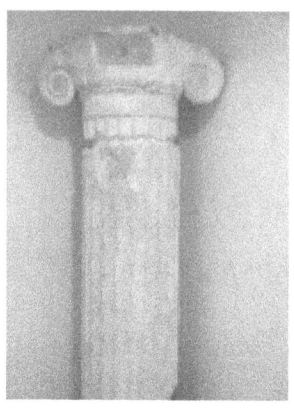

FIRST...

For the First Pillar, *Let us identify and define the God given foods that we may all enjoy as "**real food**". This would include, but is not limited to, vegetables, fruit, meat, dairy, fish, fowl, herbs, spices, nuts and organic grains. By real food I mean that it is natural, unprocessed and not modified or hybridized. I said it before, if you must open a can or package to eat, you are consuming a ton of junk (my scientific term) ☺ that your body does not need. So start by taking your canned goods, putting then in a box and labeling that box "emergency – natural disaster supplies", and put it in the bottom of your pantry.*

Now, if you're wondering what you're going to eat, just know that there is almost nothing that comes in a can that you can't make or that can't be bought fresh or frozen, but without all the additives and preservatives. Imagine good vitamin packed green beans without the excess sodium and additives (garbage) that would be packed into the cans. Fresh is best, frozen is next, and canned goods are okay for times of disaster preparedness.

I have given several suggested daily menu plans at the back of the book to assist you in knowing what to eat and/or how to begin changing the way you eat. You may follow them strictly or use them as a general guide. Note that snacks are a part of the menu plan. Do not skip them. Avoiding hunger as well as getting the vitamins and minerals you need to lose weight is important, and these snacks play an important role.

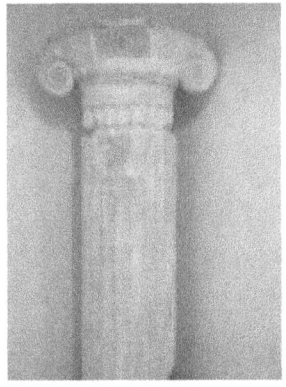

SECOND...

    For The Second Pillar, *I want you to know your junk. So that while we seem to use the term* ***"junk food"*** *often, we really do not understand just how much of our processed and modified food is really more of a "product" rather than real food. It is junk. You can consume loads of it, and actually take in very little of nutritional value, leaving your body starved for nutrients. For example, have you ever seen the label "cheese product"? Or have you ever seen the words "imitation vanilla"? These labels are telling us that the substance is a fake. It's not the real thing, but rather a product of man that is substituted for a good, wholesome product that our Creator gave us. Junk food is not just what falls out of a vending machine; it is much of what is filling our grocery store shelves. Not only will you save your money not buying these products, but you will live a healthier and longer life by taking this step. Additionally, you will have more money to buy good, organic products because of the savings you realize by not consuming all the highly processed and empty food-by-products. It is often stated that weight loss is 90% diet and 10% exercise. Many people are overweight because of what, not just how much, they eat.*

***Many people are overweight because of
what, not just how much, they eat.***

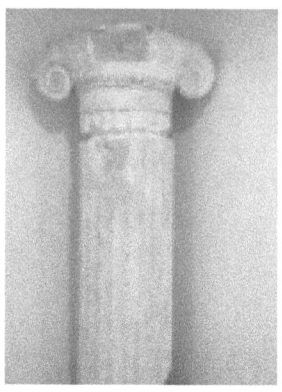

THIRD...

For The Third Pillar, *let's deal with what we drink. You are expecting me to say stop the carbonated drinks, and you should, but I'll bet you weren't thinking about dumping the juices. That's right, stop drinking fruit juices. Bottled, canned and frozen fruit juices and fruit drinks are loaded with extra sugar and other ingredients we do not need. In general, you are better off eating a piece of the fruit, say an apple, than you are in drinking a glass of apple juice. I'm not saying throw out your juicer; just understand that you don't need more than one orange worth's of juice at any given time. You wouldn't sit and eat four or five oranges at one sitting would you? Well, that's what is in a glass of fresh squeezed orange juice, minus the good fiber you want. One exception to the rule might be a homemade lemonade or limeade sweetened with stevia, which is an herbal sweetener that has been used for a thousand years.*

*The role of water is a surprise that should not be a surprise. Water plays an interesting and essential role in the lives of everyone. It is, in fact, essential for life. Water was part of God's creation as seen in Genesis 1-2. As a symbol we can understand it in terms of purification, the Spirit and life. After oxygen, water is the next most important element for sustaining life, and those who go long periods without it don't survive. But you might be interested to find that "not enough" water can also cause you problems. Dehydration and constipation are chief among the common problems we experience from not drinking enough water. I found that drinking enough water truly aided me in losing weight, so it is an important pillar in the Weigh In program. Almost without exception you will find that any plan, article or program about

weight-loss includes drinking a minimum of 8- eight oz. glasses of water. That is a start, but not enough if you want to ease constipation and lose weight. Let me suggest that you try to drink that and more. By the way, **I'm talking about water**! I know, I love my coffee too. So drink your coffee, it just doesn't count towards your water consumption. No other drinks do: not tea, not lemonade, nothing. Drink them, but get your water as well.

      WebMD says that water is one of the simplest ways to manage constipation. Let me tell you something: our society wants a pill to fix everything, but the water flows freely from the tap, so drink up.

I'll mention one more fascinating study that you may find surprising. The **International Journal of Obesity** published an Israeli study about water and obese children. It was a simple test on cold water's effect on Resting Energy Expenditure or REE. To put it simply, the REE is the energy spent while doing nothing. The results of the study showed that there was a 25% increase on the REE just by drinking cold water. This means that drinking water is helpful in weight loss and weight maintenance. Why not let water get your metabolism burning even when you're reading or watching television? So on the hour, while you work or just watch t.v., drink an 8 oz. glass of cold water.

      There is an ongoing great debate over tea and coffee. The "experts" talk about the pros and cons. Listen, both come from plants and are natural. I personally have found overwhelming studies available that speak to the health benefits of both tea and coffee in moderation. So I'm not going to add to this debate, but I will say this: enjoy your tea or coffee, just be wise if you use a sweetener or creamer, as you do not want to be drinking your calories.

***You want your metabolism
working with you,…***

      We are, as adults, made up of around 60% water! I cannot say enough about the benefits of drinking water, and no other drink can replace water. Please understand that tea, lemonade or coffee, drinks which are permitted on the **Weigh In** program, are still not a *substitute for water. Water plays a role in every kind of cellular activity in the body. Staying hydrated is vital. Your digestive system needs water. Your metabolism needs to be constantly hydrated to work at peak capacity: and you WANT your metabolism working with you, not against you.*

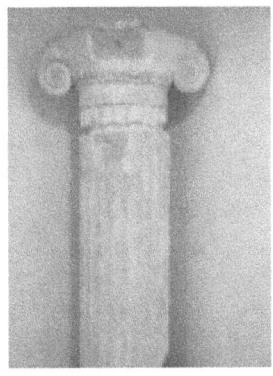

FOURTH...

The Fourth Pillar *is about logging and limiting...* **logging the good choices** *that you're making and carefully monitoring and* **limiting the foods that affect your blood glucose**, *the amount of good carbohydrates consumed daily. The program is not a low fat or fat free, it is not "high protein" or "low carb." but rather a well-rounded consumption of real foods consisting of vitamins, minerals, proteins, good fats and carbohydrates. The* **Weigh In** *program is all about making healthy choices that avoid the consumption of hybrid products like wheat, and genetically modified products like corn and soy as well as highly processed and packaged foods.*

You should be careful in your food preparation to use only good oils such as olive or coconut oil, avoid foods that drastically affect your blood sugar, and keep the good **net carbohydrates** *(See Vocabulary & Definitions) down. Be aware that the two chief culprits in hidden carbohydrates are sugar and wheat (wheat flour). Things we take for granted, like relish, chewing gum or ketchup have many hidden carbs because of sugar. Battered and fried foods are high in not-so-hidden bad carbohydrates because of the wheat batter and usually fried in* **hydrogenated oils** *(See Vocabulary & Definitions) that humans should not consume. Also, many of the "gourmet" coffees and hot chocolates we buy are more like a liquid dessert: loaded with enough bad carbs to send your blood sugar level through the roof! Buy* **organic** *fruit and vegetables when possible. Organic products help you avoid excessive pesticides as well as genetically modified organisms, which many believe are not fit for human or animal consumption: I am among those who believe this.*

While you're working to lose weight, limit fruit, leaning toward berry families: strawberries, blackberries and blueberries, about a half a cup per day. Berries are part of the "super food" groups, plus they are high in fiber, low in carbs and packed full of vitamins and minerals. In my daily meal plans I've already done the calculations for you.

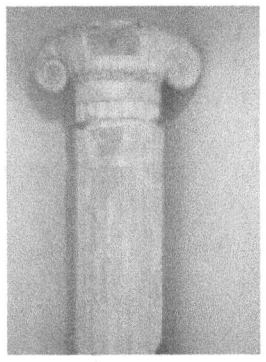

FIFTH...

The Fifth Pillar has one purpose which is getting us to move more. Most of us need to walk a little more, move a little more and/or exercise a little more. Thirty five minutes six days a week is a good goal, or every other day at the least. But you can help yourself every day by taking the stairs instead of the elevator or escalator, by not parking as close as possible when going shopping, and by simple things like mowing your lawn without using the riding mower or the power drive of the push mower. You can do leg lifts while sitting down and watching t.v., and many other low intensity exercises even while you're otherwise inactive. Exercise is as much about overall good health as it is about losing weight.

*The role of exercise. 1 Tim. 4:8 "Workouts in the gymnasium are useful..." The Message. Moderate exercise is good for us in so many ways: heart health especially. The thing is, if you use exercise alone to lose weight, the moment you stop the exercise, you stop losing and potentially start gaining weight again. Yes, exercise, just don't count on exercise alone to lose and/or maintain weight. I personally maintained my weight for years through exercise alone. I was unaware that I was doing so, but when I stopped, the weight gain began. Note: an average 10k run (6.2 miles) can burn around 1000 calories.

Research shows that moderate exercise does more for health and weight loss than extreme workouts. Yes, you can lose weight with the hardcore workouts, and you can dance it away; but when you can't work out or dance, your poor eating habits will still be there. At the same time, you must understand that exercise plays an important role in living a healthy life: don't cheat yourself by *avoiding a good walk. Remember the role of exercise and endorphins, of which I mentioned briefly in the section about keeping a sense of humor. The **Weight In** program is designed to help you strike a balance. That balance will also have a positive effect on your mood as well as your attitude. Exercise forms a fundamental part of any good health and /or weight loss program. It doesn't have to be gym membership, but you need to move. Just remember the 90% -10% rule, which bears repeating: weight loss is 90% healthy eating and 10% exercise.*

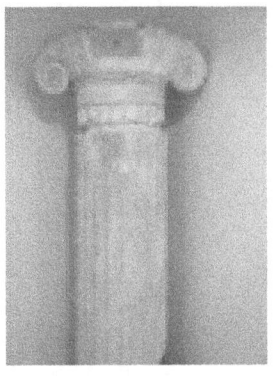

SIXTH...

The Sixth Pillar deals with **rest**. *Sleep plays an important role in our overall health as well as our weight loss or weight maintenance. Your body needs rest. Make a serious attempt to get 8 hours of sleep per day. The body needs rest to regenerate and heal. You may function okay with less, but a little more sleep will assist you in losing weight. Additionally, remember this: you're not eating while you're sleeping. ☺ Getting plenty of rest will also help lower your stress level. It is important to understand the role that rest and stress play in our bodies. Stress, in general, is not our friend. It is believed that there is a connection between stress and obesity. Cortisol.com points out that the chemical cortisol,(See Vocabulary and Definitions) triggered by stress, signals a metabolic shutdown which makes losing weight nearly impossible. Clearly, resting enough will help in lowering the stress level in your life, and will in turn assist you; at least do activities that will aide you in getting rid of your stress. Rest is one of those activities, another is found in the fifth pillar: exercise.Your body will thank you, and most likely your friends and family will too.*

While my focus in this sixth pillar is on rest, sleep in particular, don't neglect the rest that comes with a regular day off, or day of rest. An annual vacation time can be extremely beneficial as well. The biblical mandate is for mankind to rest one day out of seven, as well as have several "retreat" times per year: try it, you will not regret it. However, don't take a vacation from eating right.

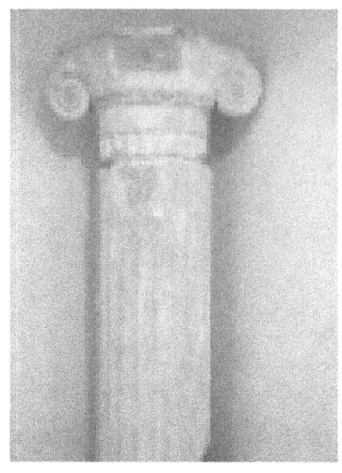

SEVENTH...

***The Seventh Pillar** is the Follow up/Maintenance plan. This pillar can and should be a celebration pillar, because once you're here, you've lost the weight. However, losing weight is one thing; keeping it off is another. Oh how I understand this, you probably do too. So **do not** skip this important seventh pillar of the **Weigh In** program, because once you have reached your goal, this final plan will help you make it a lifestyle change forever. I have simplified the seventh pillar, the follow up / maintenance plan, by giving you four rules.*

***Rule number one** in the seventh pillar is: your follow up/maintenance plan should be as long as your weight-loss plan. If you lost all your weight in three months, then your follow up / maintenance plan should be three months. If you reached your goal after one year then stick with the follow up / maintenance plan for one year. You will NEVER regret following rule number one.*

***Rule number two**: the "fake foods", those full of sugars and those highly processed are not good for you now either. Don't become a junk food or carb addict again. You are free! Stay free.*

***Rule number three**: Good things come to those who "weight". ☺ A good scale to monitor your weight is absolutely essential.*

Rule number four: *Guard against old, bad habits. +Portion control. Do not let anyone tell you that the amount of food does not matter: the portion matters. Restaurants encourage us to eat too much by selling us a portion of food that is often twice as much as we need to eat. +The Buffet. It would be much more beneficial if we would "buffet" the body and not spend time in the buffet lines! You need to understand that while we don't count calories with the* **Weigh In** *program, it is possible to consume too much, too many calories and inhibit your weight loss or maintenance. You don't need to be hungry, but you should not mistake a healthy, real food snack for a license to pig out! +A couch potato. It is not natural to be inactive. It is not good for us to avoid moving. Even in the work we do around the house, sometimes we cheat ourselves out of excellent opportunities for exercise. May I suggest that you hand wash your car; how about using a push lawnmower instead of a riding lawnmower. Be creative, but keep moving.*

*Questions and answers

Question: Is the **Weigh In** program a balanced and healthy method for weight loss?

Answer: Yes. A quick review of this method will demonstrate that an individual will take in all the necessary vitamins and minerals for good health, having no side effect except that of weight loss. In addition, the **Weigh In** program is not only good for weight loss, but as a permanent way of living. Once you reach your weight goal, you simply adjust your diet accordingly.

Question: Is constipation a problem with this method?

Answer: It can be, but not in general. Some people do experience varying levels of constipation during successful times of weight loss, primarily because the body is burning off the excess fat, which is a low grade fuel. Drinking plenty of water and eating foods rich in fiber are best, but if you don't get enough in your diet, using a mild, natural laxative like psyllium husks can alleviate this problem if it occurs. Also, cheese should be limited. It affects some people more than others, so pay attention if you are someone who gets stopped up because of cheese.

Question: Why all the nuts and seeds?

Answer: Many of the vitamins and minerals we need are found in these seeds and nuts which are loaded with vitamins, nutrients and fiber. Plus they make a really healthy snack.

Question: Won't snacking make me gain weight instead of lose?

Answer: Proper, timely snacking can be healthy and nutritious and is helpful in avoiding hunger while losing weight. You want to avoid getting ravenously hungry, and it is possible to lose weight and not be hungry all the time. Not to mention the fact that proper, healthy snacking can have a positive effect on your metabolism.

Question: Organic products are expensive. How can I afford to buy organic foods?

Answer: You will realize a huge savings when you stop buying the junk food and highly processed foods. More and more *people are waking up to this truth and are buying more carefully. So as more people buy organic the prices will continue to drop.*

Question: Do I have to take supplements? Can't I eat enough of the right foods to get the vitamins and minerals I need?

Answer: No, you do not have to take supplements. However, in the process of correcting the metabolic imbalance in your body and getting your metabolism and digestive system cranked up and working well, I have found that supplements can be of great assistance. Remember, correcting an imbalance takes more work. Also, much of the food produced today comes from mineral poor soil, so the amount of vitamins and minerals we should be getting out of our food supply is much lower than say 50 years ago.

Question: What about plateaus? I seem to be on a plateau. I'm doing everything the same, but suddenly I'm not losing weight.

Answer: This can happen to many people. It did to me. First, honestly investigate to see if you have been "cheating" just a little bit here or there. Sometimes, after a bit of success, you can get lazy, or think "a little" doesn't matter. It could also be that you're lacking in a few important vitamins and minerals. The B vitamins and Magnesium are important in your health and continued weight loss. Be sure you are getting enough food (calories) and that your body doesn't think it's starving; this is rarely the case, but you will know if it is. You can also change things up a bit. Change the exercise routine, the foods you're eating and when you're eating them. Plateaus can be discouraging, just check out the chat rooms: they're full of talk about what to do when you hit a plateaus. Be encouraged by this; that is to say, it's normal. Just shake things up a bit and stick with it!

Question: Does how I chew my food really matter?

*Answer: Yes, **chew your food adequately**. We are not good masticators, in general. We need to masticate (chew) our food more than twenty chews per bite. In an informal "survey" or shall I say observation of friends and family, I noticed that the average person was swallowing each bite after five or six chews. That is not enough! We miss out on the extraction of ALL the vitamins and minerals by not chewing our food well. Additionally, taking a little longer to chew our food allows our brain to get the message that the stomach* *is satisfied, somewhere between 15 and 20 minutes. Eating too fast and not chewing well allows us to eat beyond our need.*

Question: What about sweeteners?
Answer: I will start by stating that I do not consume white, refined sugar or
anything that contains it, and I recommend that you consider doing the same. I believe that one day we will wake up and realize that the less refined the better. That being said, I suggest you consider natural alternatives that are readily available today, like stevia or honey. FamilyDoctor.org says that stevia "Can be substituted for sugar when for baking, does not affect glucose levels, comes from an all-natural source and does not contribute to tooth decay".

Question: What about Genetically Modified Organisms (GMOs)?
Answer: Avoid them like the plague! Do not consume anything that is GMO. I hope and pray that one day these companies will not be able to sell their "cash cow" nor give it away even to third world countries. We as consumers have the power in our hands: we simply need to stop buying it. Can you tell that I feel strongly about this issue? Yes, I do. Neither animals nor humans should consume anything that has been genetically modified.

Question: What is Functional Medicine?
Answer: Basically, Functional medicine is a personalized medicine focusing on primary prevention, identification and treatment of the underlying cause rather than masking the symptoms of serious chronic disease.

Question: What is Quinoa?
Answer: While quinoa is usually considered to be a grain, it is actually a seed. Quinoa provides all 9 essential amino acids, so it is a complete protein.

Question: Does bread fall into the category of real food? I love my bread and don't see myself giving it up.
Answer: It is true that bread has become a "staple" in our society. However, wheat flour (or bread) is the chief contributor of

processed carbohydrates in our diets. I recommend that you accept the challenge to eliminate wheat flour and any products containing wheat. Just for two weeks, and see if you don't notice a difference. This made a huge difference for me in terms of allergies, mood and energy level in general.

Question: I hear a lot about "Super Foods". Is there something to this or is it all a bunch of bull?

Answer: The foods that become known as super foods do hold a great deal of nutritional value, for that reason they are called such. There are a variety of lists going around, but here are a few of the foods: black beans, lentils, blueberries, oranges, pumpkin, strawberries blackberries, broccoli, spinach, tomatoes, bell peppers, avocados, coconut oil, turkey, salmon, sardines, pecans, pistachios, walnuts, almonds, sun flower seeds, flax seed, oats, dark chocolate, olives, and brazil nuts, just to name a few.

Question: Can I really lose weight without counting calories?

*Answer: Yes and no. While the **Weigh In** program does not use calorie counting as the chief method for weight loss, it does acknowledge the generally accepted rule that one pound = 3,500 calories, more or less. However, we are all individuals, and all calories are not the same nor does the body treat all calories the same; for this reason my chief consideration is not calories.*

Question: What about alcohol like beer and wine?

Answer: This is not my area of expertise, but we all know that beer and wine tends to be loaded with carbs and sugars. One thing I do know is that there is no benefit from beer or wine that cannot be found in another non-alcoholic form.

Vocabulary & Definitions

Definitions here come from the Cambridge Dictionary available
on-line as well as other health websites.

*Anti-inflammatory: describes a drug(or herb) that is used to reduce pain and swelling.

*Antioxidant: An antioxidant is simply a molecule that prevents another molecule from oxidizing. Since there are many processes in the body which result in oxidation, the intake of antioxidants is essential to counteract some of the negative results of the buildup of too many oxidized molecules in the body. The major benefit of consuming antioxidants is that they seem to prevent and even reverse many kinds of cancer as well as heart disease and other deadly diseases.

*Carbohydrate addiction: Let me breakdown this word: Addiction - a person who has become dependent on something, especially drugs. Carbohydrate - (any of a group of) substances containing carbon, hydrogen and oxygen, especially the sugars and starches found in food.

*Constipation: unable to excrete the contents of the bowels often enough or in large enough amounts.

*Cortisol: a hormone (= a chemical made in the body).

*Dehydration: to lose water, or to cause something to lose water.

*Functional Medicine: The medical practice that focuses more on the individual and the root causes of diseases, and less on controlling diseases with medicine.

*Genetically Modified Organisms: Also known as GMOs. GMOs are crops or animals whose DNA has been altered to add traits considered desirable by producers, commonly those that help growth, like resistance to insects. GMOs make up about 90% of the corn, soybean, cotton, sugar beet and canola grown in the U.S, and the Grocery Manufacturers Association, which represents big food companies, estimates GMOs are in about 80% of packaged foods.

*Hybrid: an animal or plant produced from parents of different species or varieties.
*Hydrated: to make your body absorb water or other liquid.

*Hydrogenated oil: describes fat in foods that has had hydrogen added to it; hydrogenated fats are bad for your health.

*Hypoglycemia: a medical condition resulting from dangerously low levels of sugar in the blood.

*Insoluble fiber: Dietary fibers are found naturally in the plants we eat. They are parts of plant that do not break down in our stomachs, and instead pass through our system undigested. All dietary fibers are either soluble or insoluble. Both types of fiber are equally important for health, digestion, and preventing conditions such as heart disease, diabetes, obesity, diverticulitis, and constipation. **Insoluble fibers** are considered gut-healthy fiber because they have a laxative effect and add bulk to the diet, helping prevent constipation. These fibers do not dissolve in water, so they pass through the gastrointestinal tract fairly intact, and speed up the passage of food and waste through your gut.

*Metabolism: all the chemical processes that occur within a living thing in order to maintain life, resulting in growth and the production of energy from food.

*Net Carbohydrates: A calculation that takes the total amount of carbohydrates and subtracts the total amount of fiber, to arrive at the net count. For example: an avocado might have 12 carbs and 8 fibers, therefore it would have a net carb count of 4.

*Neurological system: relating to nerves.

*Organic: the goal of organic foods and organic farming is to "integrate cultural, biological, and mechanical practices that *foster cycling of resources, promote ecological balance, and conserve biodiversity."*

Quinoa: A whole grain like food that is actually a seed. It is an ancient food dating back to the Incas.

Refined carbohydrates: Refined carbohydrates are produced when whole plants which are high in carbohydrates are processed and stripped out of everything but the highly digestible carbohydrate (starch or sugar). This has the effect of concentrating the carb and/or breaking it down so that the body processes it very quickly, often causing a high rise in blood sugar (glycemic response). It frequently removes the fiber and most of the nutrients in the food.

Soluble fiber: attracts water and forms a gel, which slows down digestion. Soluble fiber delays the emptying of your stomach and makes you feel full, which helps control weight. Slower stomach emptying may also affect blood sugar levels and have a beneficial effect on insulin sensitivity, which may help control diabetes.

SUGGESTED MENUS

Portions are important. Try to keep meat portions to 6-8 oz. servings, (think the size of your palm). Remember that you may have coffee or tea throughout the day, but it does not count as water consumption, which is included as a reminder in the daily planner.

Here is my personal picante salsa recipe to help you spice things up. 5 medium tomatoes diced, 1 onion diced, ½ green bell pepper and ½ red bell pepper diced, 2 cloves of garlic diced, cilantro finely chopped, 1 fresh jalapeno pepper diced, and 1 sweet pepper diced, salt and pepper to taste, a dash of olive oil. (Mash all these ingredients together in the pan). Bring to a slow boil and let simmer 15 minutes. You can freely use this salsa on anything and everything you eat.

Day 1

Breakfast: Omelet – 2 eggs, ¼ cup of bell pepper, 1/8 cup of onions, ham or bacon, spinach, salt and pepper. Garnish the plate with slices of tomato and carrots cut in half down the center. Drink 16 oz. of water. Coffee or tea permitted as well, no milk or creamer, and stevia is preferred as the sweetener if needed. (7.5 carbs, 2 grams of fiber, 270 calories)

+One hour after breakfast drink a 8 oz. glass of water, or you can sip on a glass of water so long as you get enough during the day. Cold water is best.

Snack: 1 oz. of pecans, about 20 halves. Drink 16 oz. of water (1 carb., 3 grams of fiber, 180 calories) This should be about 2 hours after breakfast.

+One hour after your snack drink 8 oz. of water.

Lunch: Fish, garden salad with dark lettuce, cucumber, spinach leaves, slices of tomato, avocado, carrots, and walnuts. Use a vinegar and oil with spices dressing, or mix a tablespoon of mayo with mustard, salt and pepper. Drink 16 oz. of water. (9 carbs, 6 grams of fiber, 440 calories)

+One hour after lunch drink 8 oz. of water.

Snack: 1 oz. of natural almonds, about 25. (2 carbs, 2 grams of fiber, 160 calories) and ½ cup of blackberries, sweetened with stevia if needed. Drink 16 oz. of water. (5 carbs, 3 grams of fiber, 57 calories). This should be about 2 hours after lunch.

+One hour after your snack drink 8 oz. of water.

Dinner: Chicken, ½ cup of green beans. Garnish the plate with tomato slices with olive oil, sprinkled with salt, cilantro or oregano. Drink 16 oz. of water. (4.5 carbs, 3 grams of fiber, 372 calories)

Day 2

Breakfast: 2 eggs fried in coconut oil, a pork chop. Garnish the plate with slices of tomato and carrots cut in half down the center, ½ avocado with salt and pepper.

+One hour after your snack drink 8 oz. of water.

Snack: 1 oz. of natural almonds, about 25. Drink 16 oz. of water. (About 2 hours after breakfast)

+One hour after your snack drink 8 oz. of water.

Lunch: Chicken with onions and garlic, spinach salad with dark lettuce, cucumber, slices of tomato, avocado, carrots, and walnuts. Use a vinegar and oil with spices dressing, or mix a tablespoon of mayo with mustard, salt and pepper. Drink 16 oz. of water.

+One hour after lunch drink 8 oz. of water.

Snack: ½ cup of strawberries, 1 oz. of pecans, about 20 halves. Drink 16 oz. of water. (This should be about 2 hours after lunch).

+One hour after your snack drink 8 oz. of water.

Dinner: Steak with onions and garlic, ½ cup of squash and zucchini (fresh or grilled). Garnish the plate with tomato slices with olive oil, then sprinkled with salt, cilantro or oregano. Drink 16 oz of water.

Day 3

Breakfast: Two boiled eggs, ¼ cup of blueberries, ¼ cup of raspberries, and 1 oz. of walnuts. Drink 16 oz. of water.

+One hour after your breakfast drink 8 oz. of water.

Snack: 1 oz. of pumpkin seeds, 1 celery stick with 2 teaspoons of organic peanut butter, Drink 16 oz. of water.

+One hour after your snack drink 8 oz. of water.

Lunch: Turkey breast with your choice of spices, ½ cup of broccoli (fresh or grilled), garnish the plate with sliced cucumbers with olive oil salt and pepper, cilantro or oregano.

+One hour after your lunch drink 8 oz. of water.

Snack: 1 oz. of natural, roasted sunflower seeds, 1 boiled egg.

+One hour your snack drink 8 oz. of water.

Dinner: Chicken wraps with picante salsa. This is boiled or grilled chicken wrapped in dark lettuce leaves or cabbage leaves if you prefer. Add spices to your liking and shoot for three. Think of this as fajitas but with something healthy. ½ cup of your choice of veggies. Drink 16 oz. of water.

Make your own menus

    A breakfast substitute: True whole grain toast with peanut butter, one fruit of choice. A lunch substitute: Choice of vegetable, venison or lamb, green salad.

    A snack substitute: Choice of nuts, blueberries or another berry family. A dinner substitute: Zucchini or squash noodles, tomato sauce and beef (or venison) with your favorite spices, serve just like spaghetti. Any non-processed meat is a good choice alongside a vegetable and green salad with a healthy dressing. Remember to use your spices freely. Avoid a rut, that is, doing the same thing meal after meal: change it up.

FINAL THOUGHTS

We are fearfully and wonderfully created. Our bodies are just amazing! When we take care of what we have been given, or when we work to recover that which we have lost (or misplaced) the result will be a happier and healthier life.

Today I think more about the good habits I have adopted in my life as well as the good example I have set for family and friends. I also know that instead of shortening my life with destructive habits, I have opened up the possibilities of living a longer, healthier and joyful life.

People look at me and think, "If he can do it, so can I". And they are correct! Listen to me: you can do it!

So I leave you with this to think on: There is a Great Physician who has provided what we need to live long, healthy lives. He has seven assistant physicians; they are called:

**Fresh air,
water,
sunshine,
rest,
a diet filled with real food,
exercise and
laughter.**

Bibliography

Family Doctor.org-

Health Guidance.org –

The International Journal of Obesity: Israeli Study –

The Message (The Bible)-

USDA -

WebMD on line –

Weston Price & Vitamin A @WestonPrice.org -

About the Author

Mark lets people know right up front that he is not a doctor. It is clear, however, that his research, experience and success in losing weight and maintaining weight loss demonstrate that he does indeed have a good grasp on health and good nutrition well beyond that of average laymen in these fields.

It may well be that Mark's ability to explain things in these laymen's terms is what has caused people to ask him to share his story and how they can do the same.

Mark is married to his high school sweetheart, Kelly. They have two adult children and two grandchildren.

Mark and Kelly are Ordained Ministers; Kelly, his wife is also a Licensed Midwife, and they work as Missionaries just off the Northwest coast of Africa. Mark has a Bachelor of Arts Degree in Bible and Theology and is currently working on a Master's Degree. He likes to study nutrition and fitness, both formally and informally.

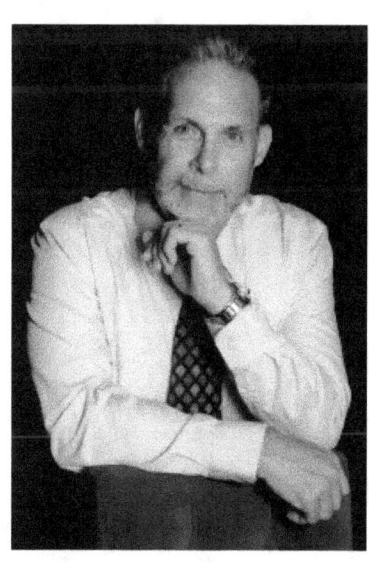

www.ingramcontent.com/pod-product-compliance
Lightning Source LLC
Chambersburg PA
CBHW070841290526
45795CB00002B/943